Being a Solo Librarian in H

CHANDOS
INFORMATION PROFESSIONAL SERIES
Series Editor: Ruth Rikowski
(email: Rikowskigr@aol.com)

Chandos' new series of books is aimed at the busy information professional. They have been specially commissioned to provide the reader with an authoritative view of current thinking. They are designed to provide easy-to-read and (most importantly) practical coverage of topics that are of interest to librarians and other information professionals. If you would like a full listing of current and forthcoming titles, please visit www.chandospublishing.com.

New authors: we are always pleased to receive ideas for new titles; if you would like to write a book for Chandos, please contact Dr Glyn Jones on g.jones.2@elsevier.com or telephone +44 (0) 1865 843000.

Being a Solo Librarian in Healthcare

Pivoting for 21st Century Healthcare Information Delivery

Elizabeth Burns, MLS

ELSEVIER

AMSTERDAM • BOSTON • HEIDELBERG • LONDON
NEW YORK • OXFORD • PARIS • SAN DIEGO
SAN FRANCISCO • SINGAPORE • SYDNEY • TOKYO
Chandos is an imprint of Elsevier

CP
CHANDOS
PUBLISHING

Chandos Publishing is an imprint of Elsevier
225 Wyman Street, Waltham, MA 02451, USA
Langford Lane, Kidlington, OX5 1GB, UK

ISBN: 978-0-08-100122-6

British Library Cataloguing-in-Publication Data
A catalogue record for this book is available from the British Library

Library of Congress Cataloging-in-Publication Data
A catalog record for this book is available from the Library of Congress

Library of Congress Control Number: 2015939544

For information on all Chandos publications
visit our website at http://store.elsevier.com/

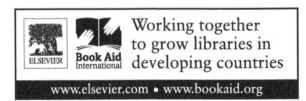

Working together
to grow libraries in
developing countries

www.elsevier.com • www.bookaid.org

This book is dedicated
to all the healthcare librarians,
especially hospital librarians.
No finer bouquet of people.

Contents

About the author

Elizabeth Burns is currently a Medical Librarian at the Kansas City Veterans Affairs Medical Center in Kansas City, MO. She is a member of the Medical Library Association (MLA), the Mid-Continent Medical Library Association (MCMLA), and the Health Sciences Library Network of Kansas City (HSLNKC).

In 2006, she received the HSLNKC award for Outstanding One-Person Health Science Library. She was presented the Barbara McDowell Award for Excellence in Hospital Librarianship in 2009. This award was established in 1984 in honor of Barbara McDowell, Chief of Library Services in Sioux Falls, South Dakota. Nominees are judged on Hospital Library leadership/innovation, Local group participation/leadership, Chapter participation/leadership, and National participation/leadership.

She has presented at MLA and has served on various committees in the HSLNKC group and MCMLA. In particular, she was a member of the MCMLA Library Advocacy Committee and then was Chair of the committee from 2010 to 2013.

Preface

Initially, I was asked to write a textbook on solo-librarianship in healthcare. I intended the book to be an introduction to the different duties of a Medical Librarian. However, as I began mapping it out and researching the literature, the book gradually became more of a revealing of the current atmosphere for healthcare librarians. My many years of serving on the MCMLA Library Advocacy Committee had given me contact with librarians whose libraries had been eliminated. We wrote letters to hospital administrators and had meetings discussing what could be done, but hospital libraries continued to be closed. Obviously, I couldn't write a textbook and ignore the elephant in the room.

So, what started out as an introduction to healthcare solo-librarianship, became a kind of litany for hospital librarians and a call for common sense. I have no idea whether this small book will make any difference to the current tide of closing hospital libraries. I am one small voice, but I hope I am speaking well for the many wonderful, intelligent healthcare librarians I have met over the years and for the hospital staff who could sure use the help of a librarian.

Elizabeth Burns

Acknowledgments

I wish to thank George and Harriet at Chandos Publishing for accepting and liking my skimpy book when they were expecting a textbook with many more pages.

Forethoughts

The title of this book chooses the words solo healthcare librarian to bring attention to the dwindling number of medical librarians at a time when they are needed more than ever. I hope to show that today's medical librarian can contribute to improving patient care, but is not being utilized and in some hospitals, no longer exists. This book is written for the stakeholders in healthcare and for anyone considering healthcare librarianship as a profession.

When I began organizing my thoughts for this book, I did a mind map. Some people will know exactly what I'm talking about. For those who don't, mind mapping is a way of linking ideas. It is a way of connecting thoughts which leads to discovering the major ideas, and how these connect with other subsidiary subject matter. The major focus of the mind map was to get a clear idea of what constitutes the best representation of what a medical librarian does. Healthcare librarians provide information storage, information retrieval, and information delivery. As I jotted down the many duties of the solo librarian, the mind map took on the shape of two circles or wheels. The hub of one wheel was library patron needs, and the other, librarian needs. The many other ideas were like spokes radiating out from these two hubs, with much overlapping. The image of these two wheels brought to mind a bicycle, but then a third hub began to form, which had to do with elements that kept the other two balanced and running smoothly. These other elements or what I would call core requirements came from a poll I sent to the MedLib Listserv. The MedLib listserv is a public discussion list for medical and health science librarians. The question posed was "What is the one piece of advice you would give to a librarian who has to do it all alone? Or, what is something helpful to make the job easier or more efficient?" The answers were varied, but these four dominated.

1. Flexibility or the ability to multitask and prioritize
2. Networking
3. Supportive boss
4. Volunteers.

These four topics formed the third hub bringing to my mind a triangular image or a wheelbarrow. Being a person who loves to play with symbols, I looked in the Penguin Dictionary of Symbols (1996) and discovered the wheelbarrow actually makes a fitting ideogram for an information delivery system, of which librarians are only a part:

> *The symbolism of the wheelbarrow derives from an overall view of the object regarded as an extension of the human arm and as a miniature farm-cart. In fact it symbolizes the enhancement of human strength in three different ways. The first is in intensity, since the two handles of the wheelbarrow form levers; the second in volume through the capacity of the barrow; and the third in freedom of movement, thanks to the wheel. . . Its balance also depends on the person holding the handles and it is just as easy to tip it over as it is to push it forward. In this context it might stand for fate with all its potential and all its ambivalence (p. 1104).*

Further support for this symbol came from the Janet Doe Lecture given by Margaret Bandy at the 2014 MLA (Medical Library Association) Conference in Chicago. Margaret spoke about pivoting as a word to describe quickly adapting to change and moving librarianship to interdisciplinary collaboration. She spoke about pivoting as a way of changing the trajectory of the profession. As I listened, the wheelbarrow image came to mind again. A wheelbarrow pivots very well, and it can be filled with all sorts of things. I began to see the wheelbarrow as an icon for an information delivery system for all healthcare. If you think this is too antiquated an image, I would argue that perhaps today this is exactly what we need to counter the blown-out-of proportion misinformation circulating about the Internet. It was with the advent of the Internet that everyone believed all information would be available and free. Sometimes I think this one idea is responsible for doctors and residents using Google and not using the library purchased databases. We all know that the databases that hospitals pay thousands of dollars to search are far from free. We also know that with this misperception of the internet came the idea that librarians and libraries were no longer needed. Ironically, librarians were early adopters of computers and the Internet. For a quick look at the last 35 years in librarianship, see Dudden (2004). It is the public perception of librarians that is outdated. The wheelbarrow may represent a need to return to commonsense, to a grounding on what works for a twenty-first century information delivery system. The wheelbarrow is a working person's tool, and some things are so basic, they are timeless.

Of course, here we are considering the fate of healthcare libraries and librarians. Will hospital libraries exist 10 years from now? Will clinical librarianship or informationists embedded in different departments replace the healthcare librarian and library? Who or what is responsible for the direction of libraries moving toward the future? Solo librarians are acutely aware of the precarious circumstances surrounding medical libraries. Nationwide, all of us have witnessed many hospital library closings. In an effort to stem the tide, the MLA set up a task force to investigate and come up with ways to help hospital libraries. The National Network of Libraries of Medicine (NNLM) and the Mid-Continent Medical Library Association (MCMLA) Library Advocacy Committee composed letters to send to administrators, detailing a list of reasons for keeping the libraries and librarians. It soon became evident the letters were too little, too late. Though librarians are passionate about the profession and do publish excellent articles on the many services provided, we've been mainly publishing in library related journals. In other words, we were preaching to the choir. Shumaker (2012) agrees, saying, "Medical librarians have done amazing work, but it's all written up in the medical library journals, and if you're not a medical librarian reading those journals, you probably haven't read about it" (xv). Therefore, I think the title of this book almost begs for a subtitle such as "A book not written for librarians" or "Healthcare librarians need not read this book." A librarian friend of mine shared this with me and I'm sure there are many stories similar to this one. She said that a friend of hers, who is a pharmacist was in the library with another pharmacist who commented "She's got the best job in the hospital. All she has to do is check out books to people." Healthcare librarians encounter this misperception, often. What does a solo librarian do? Everything in the wheelbarrow. That's what this book will cover. The focus will mainly be on the major services, but also how these services collide with other seen and unseen forces.

The three hubs: the patron's needs, the solo librarian's needs, and the core requirements obtained from the poll intermingle creating an iterative quality to the content of this book. The core requirements help to support and balance, allowing pivoting as the solo librarian performs daily work. However, when we talk about pivoting, there is a more far-reaching scale of pivoting that this book will address. In this information-rich world, librarians have the potential and the obligation to serve in ways that will alter and improve delivery of healthcare. I hope that this glimpse of healthcare librarianship will contribute to rousing all stakeholders involved in improving diagnosis and treatment of patients.

Before moving to Chapter 2, I want to say a few words about flexibility and multitasking. I think I prefer the word flexibility rather than multitasking. Flexibility is moving from one job to another and then returning to the task that was temporarily suspended. Multitasking gives one the impression of doing several jobs at the same time and perhaps not a good idea. For example, doing a literature search requires deep concentration and is almost impossible to do simultaneously with other work. Even though I've heard that the Millennial is the master of multitasking, I think even a Millennial or Net Gener would have to do some reflecting while conducting a search. In addition, whatever task you are engaged in, it sometimes helps to keep a note pad close by to jot down reminders as you find yourself pulled in so many directions. You want to be flexible, not scatterbrained. Flexibility means that when that patron or patient enters the library, you are ready and willing to listen to their need for information. It could be a request for a book, a journal article, a literature search, or perhaps they don't know where they can find what they need. A solo librarian is never bored. With such a variety of duties to perform, an important part of a solo librarian's job is prioritizing. Usually, the list runs like this, as to what work gets done first.

1. Literature searches for urgent patient care
2. Other literature searches
3. Filling requests for journal articles
4. Everything else.

This book is meant to be an introduction to medical librarianship through the eyes of a solo librarian. This is not a "how to" book. There are many books that focus on the various responsibilities of medical librarianship. Therefore, you will not find instructions on how to catalog. This is covered when you earn a Masters in Library Science. What you will encounter in this book is a glimpse of the current atmosphere of Healthcare Librarianship, which is in dynamic flux at this time. This is not a profession for the faint-hearted.

As a healthcare solo librarian, it is important to be aware of the milieu in which evidence-based medicine resides. Throughout this book, I will use EB as an abbreviation for evidence-based medicine or evidence-based practice. Chapter 2 will discuss literature searches and EB, but even more important, the barriers to practicing EB. Teaching and information/document delivery will also be included as core services. Chapter 3 covers purchasing and marketing, which requires a librarian who is steeped in the constantly changing publishing environment. Chapter 4 looks at the cycle of maintaining electronic resources, also requiring skills and knowledge usually learned on the job and taking time. Chapter 5 shows the importance of networking and the different forms of support for the solo librarian. Chapter 6 is a brief synopsis of thoughts on the content of this book.

Bedrock services

2

Chapter Outline Head

Literature searches

As already noted, literature searches take first priority. This means that no matter what you are working on, if a request comes for a search, you suspend your task and do the search. Time is of the essence. As a healthcare librarian, you will know where to search and you will develop a skill in knowing when it is ok to stop searching. Now, hopefully, there are some readers who do not know what a literature search is.

A literature search is a request from a patron for healthcare information. The patron's question is usually regarding diagnosis, therapy, prognosis, or perhaps prevention. There is an art to asking the patron what information they would like to have, or what librarians call the reference interview. This is another topic covered in graduate school. The librarian's skill lies in knowing which database to search and knowing how to search in a particular database. One of the best known databases is Medline, housed in PubMed, from the National Institute of Health and the National Library of Medicine. It is available for free on the Internet at http://www.ncbi.nlm.nih.gov/pubmed. Medline/PubMed provides mainly citations and abstracts of articles, and some full-text, but not as much as contained in commercial databases. Commercial databases can range in price from a few thousand dollars to over one hundred thousand dollars. The medical librarian has a budget and carefully weighs the pros and cons of where to spend the money, but more on this in Chapter 3. Our focus is on the literature search which can be simple or complex. For example, you might be asked to find articles that address nursing night shift workers and their quality of life, hospital discharge practices, best practices for wound care, hospital readmission reduction programs, perioperative device management, or the safety and effectiveness of a particular medication. It is gratifying to find the information that answers the question or provides support for the decision making process of the healthcare worker. Depending on the subject matter of the search and the complexity, you could be delivering articles via email to the doctor or nurse within 10–15 minutes or for more complex searches, perhaps an hour or more. The hospital librarian searches on a daily basis and offers this service to the patron, which ultimately means the doctor makes a more informed decision.

Evidence-based practice (EB)

As a healthcare librarian, you will become familiar with Evidence-Based Practice, sometimes called Evidence-Based Medicine and abbreviated in this book as EB. Probably, the most famous of the founders and promoters of EB are David Sackett and Gordon Guyatt, who authored some excellent books. Sackett (2000) gives this definition: "Evidence-based medicine (EBM) is the integration of best research evidence with clinical expertise and patient values." EB is not just about the literature. It includes the doctor's expertise, consulting with colleagues, and takes into consideration the patient's concerns.

There is another form of EB that needs mention. In 2003, in an effort to improve the U.S. healthcare system, the Medicare Modernization Act (MMA) authorized the Agency for Healthcare Research and Quality (AHRQ) to research the effectiveness of medical treatments through CER (Tanenbaum, 2008). CER stands for comparative effectiveness research. It is a form of EB, but where EB's gold standard is the randomized controlled trial (RCT), CER chooses to focus on comparing different treatments to find the best in particular cases or patients with comorbidities. An RCT looks at efficacy, or the power to produce a result, and CER looks at effectiveness or something that works (Tanenbaum, 2008). The Institute of Medicine (IOM) created a list of prioritized topics for CER to research. The list is available online at http://www.iom. edu/Reports/2009/ComparativeEffectivenessResearchPriorities.aspx.

Even though CER appears to be a more realistic approach, there are some concerns as to who and what will define and determine the best or most effective care, as there are multiple points of view to consider such as comorbidities, underlying risk, adherence to therapies, disease stage and severity, insurance coverage and demographics (Eden, Wheatley, McNeil, & Sox, 2008).

There are many reasons for promoting EB. We could begin with diagnostic errors.

According to an article in the British Medical Journal on Quality and Safety, at least 1 in 20 US adults or approximately 12 million adults each year are affected by diagnostic errors and that about half of these errors could potentially be harmful (Singh, Meyer, & Thomas, 2014). A 2009 article in *Journal of the American Medical Association (JAMA)* gives this definition of diagnostic error:

> *Diagnostic error can be defined as a diagnosis that is missed, wrong, or delayed, as detected by some subsequent definitive test or finding. However, not all misdiagnoses result in harm, and harm may be due to either disease or intervention. Misdiagnosis-related harm can be defined as preventable harm that results from the delay or failure to treat a condition actually present (when the working diagnosis was wrong or unknown) or from treatment provided for a condition not actually present.*
> *(Newman-Toker & Pronovost, 2009, p. 1060)*

A 2014 article titled "The Next Organizational Challenge: Finding and Addressing Diagnostic Error" in the *Joint Commission Journal on Quality and Patient Safety* estimates the death toll from diagnostic errors in the United States at 40,000 to 80,000 per year (Graber et al., 2014). Furthermore, diagnostic errors are costly. Hospital readmissions and unwarranted treatments given are unnecessary expenses. Patient safety and quality of care are two of the reasons EB is being promoted today.

The Joint Commission recognizes the importance of access to information and established the IM.5.10 standard that requires healthcare organizations to provide the means for healthcare professionals to access information in print, electronic, and audio formats, day or night. There is no requirement to have a library on site, but only that there is a contractual agreement in place with some library. This agreement is not always a favorable contract for the hospital without a library and librarian, but more on this topic later when we look at purchasing and licensing.

Given that all healthcare organizations strive for safety and the best care possible, and that the Joint Commission promotes keeping up with medical information, one might assume physicians and all healthcare staff need only keep up with the published literature. Of course, this is easier said than done. Let's consider the barriers to practicing EB, doctors' perceptions of EB, lack of search skills and lack of time, and lack of funds to support EB practice.

Barriers to practicing EB

Doctors' and residents' perception of EB

Recently, the IOM published its report on the governance and financing of graduate medical education (GME). Comments about this report came from David Asch in the *New England Journal of Medicine (NEJM)*. Asch (2014) noted the lack of research in medical education in contrast to the sustained support for biomedical research. He says "the current duration, settings, and organization of GME are more the product of tradition than of evidence and have changed little in the face of substantial changes in the health needs of patients and the systems for delivering care."

The literature presents a complex situation when it comes to doctors not embracing EB practice. A systematic review revealed major barriers which included, mindset, EB competencies, and professional group norms (Swennen, 2013). As a librarian, you should be aware of these barriers so that you can more consciously provide service that will facilitate EB for the doctor or healthcare worker. Let's look at the mindsets and group norms.

Swennen (2013) reveals that EB generates some fears or discomfort in the minds of physicians and residents. Swennen shows that it is not just a lack of time that keeps doctors and residents from practicing EB. Some doctors see EB as not recognizing their expertise and fear losing their autonomy. There is also a strong hierarchical order among doctors and residents making residents reluctant to challenge the established norms of practice (Swennen, 2013). van Dijk (2010) likewise says that there is fear of repercussions from staff when confronting them with new evidence and that "preferences of the clinical supervisors may also influence the practice of the resident" (p. 1163). Swennen (2013) calls it "an 'expert-based' pecking order and nonreciprocal communication" (p. 3). Green (2000) agrees with this assessment noting that internal medicine residents encounter two questions for every three patients, but only pursue 29% of their questions. Another barrier voiced by residents is a lack of computers available at the point of care with a patient. However, as a further testament to the strong influence of the hospital culture barrier, one resident stated "Don't drop laptops in our laps and then think we're going to change over-night" (Green, 2005, p. 181). Given that the hospital culture is a formidable barrier to EB practice, Green (2005) proposes a stronger advocacy for EB educational programs in the hospital's mission, but even this may not be enough.

Clinicians' lack of time and lack of skills

Zipperer (2004) notes that access to medical literature has changed dramatically and that clinicians do their own research if time and skills permit, but that this is not often the case. Studies show that 59% of clinicians "experience difficulty navigating or searching for medical information" (Bennett, 2005, p. 3). Dhaliwal (2013) writes that the greatest barrier to point-of-care-learning (POCL) is lack of time, along with information overload and case complexity. Likewise, van Dijk (2010) and Green (2005) speak of the lack of time and lack of skills as barriers to EB practice.

Between 1865 and 2006, the Index Medicus, which is what librarians searched before Medline, grew from 1600 references to nearly 10 million (Bastian, 2010). In the 1970s and 1980s systematic reviews appeared as a way to review and make sense of the literature. Today there are systematic reviews of systematic reviews. Bastian (2010) writes that back in 1979 there were about 14 trials a day being published. Thirty years later there are 11 systematic reviews and 75 trials being published daily. There are also numerous unpublished reports from conferences and organizations that librarians refer to as grey literature.

> *To ask why we need libraries at all, when there is so much information available elsewhere, is about as sensible as asking if roadmaps are necessary now that there are so very many roads.*
> *Jon Bing, Professor of Information Technology Law,*
> *University of Oslo, Norway.*

The above quote causes me to think that instead of a Masters in Library Science (MLS), the healthcare librarian should have a GPS listed after his or her name. Sorry, couldn't resist. In addition to the increase in publications, there are a number of databases and each with a different design for searching. In 2000, Davidoff wrote that considering the necessary skills needed for searching the literature, a doctor can easily take an hour and that a physician will never have that kind of time and that it is no wonder that doctors prefer to consult their colleagues when they have questions. Davidoff (2000) sees this as fine, if the colleagues are well grounded in published evidence. Likewise, Swennen (2013), van Dijik (2010), and Green (2005) detect a cultural and attitudinal barrier. Davidoff sees doctors as not wanting to be seen as needing help. In the current information environment, Davidoff (2000) says that it makes no sense for doctors to do their own information retrieval in the same way it would be ridiculous for them to perform all their own clinical lab work and computed tomography. It appears that Davidoff has been writing on the topic of utilizing clinical librarians for many years and though it might appear that not much has changed, he points out that probably the best way to bring about change is through pilot programs, of which there have been many. David Shumaker's book *The Embedded Librarian* is an excellent source for the forces driving clinical librarianship. It covers several studies of embedded librarians who work as clinical librarians in healthcare teams. He notes that the idea began in the 1960s when the practice of medicine was being seen as a team activity. According to Eden (2008), "The era of physician as sole healthcare decision maker is long past. In today's world, healthcare decisions are made by multiple people, individually or in collaboration, in multiple contexts for multiple purposes."

Lack of money versus high cost of not finding information

Davidoff (2011) makes the point that the United States pays billions of dollars for millions of unnecessary clinical tests when it might improve care and save money by funding medical libraries and librarians. He states that the budgetary constraints or "perverse priorities" have resulted in the complete elimination of many hospitals' medical libraries in an effort to "cut costs." Furthermore, the Patient Protection and Affordable Care Act includes no provision for improving clinical information delivery to those who make medical decisions and that "It is time to build a medical information delivery system worthy of the medical profession" (p. 1907, 2011).

To ignore the need for a better way of delivering information to the right person at the right time is dangerous and expensive. Feldman (2004) speaks about several incidents or information disasters. She notes that information disasters are caused "not by lack of information, but rather by not connecting the right information to the right people at the right time" (p. 3). Furthermore, "We need to embed both people and information within a system that fits how people in the organization work, that understands the workflow and when the needs for information arise" (p. 4). When a hospital closes the library and no longer has a librarian, there is harm done to the operations of the hospital. Equally bad is when a hospital replaces the librarian with a clerk or someone who has no knowledge of Library Science or medical resources. It is both comical and sad to read a post on the MedLib Listserv from a person who has been hired to replace the librarian. The nonlibrarian is asking which "magazines" she should buy for the library and asks if there are any online resources that would be helpful.

As a solo healthcare librarian, it will be almost impossible to spend a significant part of your day embedded in another department. If the library was funded properly, you would not be a solo librarian and would be able to spend a good amount of time going on rounds or attending Morning Report with doctors and/or nurses. Without the funds, the solo librarian must network with other healthcare workers within the hospital in order to find out where your services are needed. We will look into this later when we discuss networking. I want to return to Davidoff's vision of an information delivery system.

Speaking about clinical library programs, Davidoff (2011) writes that only about 12% of Canadian and U.S. Medical Libraries deliver information this way. Of course, there are probably more clinical librarians today. However, we still continue to see library closings with no other delivery system to replace the librarian. Setting up an improved information service doesn't have to transition into an embedded informationist. One particular study comes to mind. Dhaliwal (2011) refers to this study when he says "Medical librarians are far more adept at navigating the entire canon of medical knowledge than are physicians, but their skills have not been leveraged for POCL." He then refers to a study where a librarian was utilized as a POCL resource. This study was an RCT where the average time for the librarian to provide needed information was 13.68 minutes (McGowan, 2008). This just-in-time service, or JIT librarian service, decreased return patient visits, referrals, and costs. The study also showed a cost savings based on the difference in salaries of librarians versus doctors and the time spent searching with physicians taking a longer time. The JIT librarian brings to mind Toyota Lean methods and Six Sigma. Any Google search will bring up information on Lean and Six Sigma methodology. Toyota Lean lists different types of waste and Six Sigma added the waste of unused human talent or underutilizing a person's capabilities. It is wasteful not to have librarians as part of the healthcare team.

There have been many studies reported, usually in library journals, on the benefits of engaging the help of librarians in healthcare. One particular study warrants mention. It comes from the book *Evidence-Based Librarianship: Case Studies and Active Learning Exercises* (Connor, 2007). Healthcare librarians at the Louisiana State University Health Sciences Center (LSU) in Shreveport partnered with the Internal Medicine physicians during the morning report. At the end of the hour, doctors presented questions based on the data presented. The librarian conducted a search to find literature to answer the questions. The results of this collaboration are nicely plotted out in graphs, but for the sake of brevity, suffice it to say that the length of stay (LOS) was significantly less for the morning report patients than for the comparison group patients and there were significant savings for the hospital. This scenario demonstrates not only savings for the hospital but also education for the doctors and residents.

Of course, there is the ground-breaking program at Johns Hopkins Welch Library. I remember reading the article in *USA Today* talking about the librarians being transformed into "e-sherpas" (Kolowich, 2010). Today, the program has expanded to the point that the Welch Library is no longer needed as a central location for the librarians. The informationists are embedded in various departments, making it easier for the librarian to know what staff really need. Must healthcare librarians everywhere be transformed into informationists? Perhaps, perhaps not. A solo healthcare librarian can still deliver cost-saving information to clinical staff without having to be stationed outside of the library.

Zipperer (2010) explores ways the librarian can contribute by being available at the point of need. She proposes being proactive. Rather than waiting for hospital administrators to sanction a program, she lists ways to reach out and partner with other clinical staff. Like doctors, nurses lack the time needed for keeping up with the deluge of EB literature. Maatta and Wallmyr (2010) present a study where two clinical librarians took a more active role with nurses. They participated on rounds, handovers, and other parts of a nurse's daily duties. The librarians discovered the nurses were frustrated because they wanted to have time for EB, but that their job was "jammed with many tasks to be performed quickly" (p. 3430). They were authorized to take time for this, but it was difficult to find the time. One important topic that came up was that EB ". . . may also be a way for nurses to get authority and confidence to articulate nursing caring issues" (Maatta & Wallmyr, 2010).

As discussed earlier, diagnostic error is a huge problem in the United States. Using a librarian could contribute to decreasing diagnostic error. The name or title we give ourselves shouldn't matter. Most librarians are capable of working with residents and clinical teams. Embedded clinical librarians or informationists, or standard medical librarians are not just for the Johns Hopkins hospitals, but should be for all healthcare institutions. Patients should be given the best care everywhere.

Teaching and training

In July 2014, the IOM released its report on financing GME. Rovner (2014) commenting on the IOM report makes the point that the federal government provides more than $11 billion per year for training of doctors. The question she poses is how this money contributes to the medical workforce we need in the twenty-first century? One might propose teaching the residents how to search as a way to improve the workforce, but as discussed earlier, the doctors already have enough on their plates and would rather search Google or consult their colleagues.

Teaching hospital staff how to find the information they need is important, but even more important and more basic is helping them discover that the library resources are relevant to their work. You could say it is a wheelbarrow basic. Residents, in particular, tend to use Google for all of their searching needs. The pervasive climate is the belief that the information is readily out there on the internet and if you can't find it, then you aren't internet savvy. The following is a good example of how teaching could be conducted in hospitals across the country.

Weaver (2011) shares an account of how medical librarians created a "teaching package" for the residents in a children's hospital in Colorado. Use of the small library had declined for several years, so the librarians decided to choose a particular group and tailor services to their needs. In 2001, after speaking to the head of the GME and the residency coordinator, one of the librarians was allowed to attend the Morning Report twice a week. The librarian took notes and after the Morning Report, spoke with the chief resident to discuss the types of information that would be helpful for the residents. In the beginning, there was a lack of dissemination of the material that the librarian sent to the chief resident, but eventually the chief resident created an email list. Consequently, a learning package was created containing a written record of the case, written by the chief resident and also the librarian's links to full-text articles. This learning package was a big success and the librarian was now attending Morning Rounds 5 days a week. Clinicians who sometimes couldn't attend the Morning Report were able to receive the learning package via email. Soon, other allied health workers heard of this and asked to be included on the list. The list grew to include interns, attending physicians, Corporate Compliance people, nurses, the risk manager, and more. Even the residents who graduated and moved on, asked to remain on the list. One unexpected result was that people on the list started exploring and using the library resources. Also, there was more traffic in the library as residents and others came to use the computers and books. This example of partnering in educating residents needs support in order to become a nationwide practice.

Traditional teaching can take place in a classroom or can be a one on one partnering. There are theories and methodologies on how to teach people to search. If the reader is interested in this profession, you will need to take classes yourself on searching and at the same time observe what works well. There are classes available at conferences and periodically online through the National Network of Libraries of Medicine (NNLM). PubMed also provides online tutorials. It is advisable to become familiar with Medline/ PubMed because one never knows which commercial database will be available at the hospital where you work next.

Though some PubMed classes can be an all-day event, you will probably have to restrict your class to 1 hour. The hour should include some lecture, but an equal or more amount of time for interactive lessons where people can pair up in twos or threes to search and share their approaches. Ideally, everyone would be interested in learning searching techniques and love it. In reality, librarians know that some people would prefer that you do a search for them or at least a mediated search.

Doing a search with the nurse or clinician is sometimes the best way to teach. They have the background knowledge and you have the searching skills. It's also a learning experience for you as they share their clinical knowledge with you. Partnering is a great way to empower them and show them sometimes intricate steps involved.

Information and document delivery

Healthcare librarians teach patrons where they can access articles in the electronic online journals and databases. Nevertheless, more often than not, patrons will request journal articles from the librarian. I think most librarians don't mind filling these requests because they know healthcare workers have busy schedules and don't have time, and it is just faster to have the librarian locate the literature. You will fill many requests every day. It is very important to do these as quickly as possible. Speed is everything. This is a service that can make the patron's job less stressful. Sometimes you will get long lists of articles from someone who is conducting research. There is no need to deliver all of them in 1 day, but do them in a timely manner.

Docline is the Medical Librarian's online interlibrary loan database, coming from the National Library of Medicine and the National Institute of Health. All medical librarians use it to request interlibrary loans. A hospital must have a library with books and journals in order to reciprocate and participate in interlibrary loaning. The librarian can set up a routing table, which contains a list of libraries that requests will be routed to. This routing table must be updated regularly. There are ways to search in Docline to find a book and request only one chapter. There are ways to find a library that owns a journal title that is not listed in PubMed. Overall, Docline is an excellent resource.

Another much researched form of information is the clinical decision support system or CDSS. The CDSS is usually housed in the electronic health record or EHR. Cimino (2013) and others have made significant advances in the development of CDSSs. This is another area where Medical librarians could help. For example, in the creation and maintenance of the "Infobuttons." Infobuttons are the links to medical information resources. Cimino (2013) states that decisions about which information resources should be linked to, requires people who understand the institution's users and information needs. I would suggest a medical librarian would have current and in-depth knowledge of electronic resources and which ones would be most appropriate for a particular subject. Also, because guidelines depend upon current, authoritative information sources, the librarian is well situated to alerting the EHR team about newly published literature and reports. In addition, librarians know how to set up searches in the NCBI section of PubMed that would automatically send via email, any new literature published on particular topics. The searches could be tailored to specific limits, such as age of patient, comorbidities, specific medications, and more. These emails could be set to deliver daily, weekly, or monthly.

Purchasing

3

Chapter Outline Head

Book purchasing

Printed books are still needed by physicians, nurses, and other allied health staff. In addition, regulatory agencies such as the Joint Commission mandate that hospitals have backup core print resources in the event of a power outage, server problems, or any other malfunction. Even without a crisis situation, the library needs to provide some print resources. Even though there is a plethora of published journal literature, there are some questions that can only be answered by a textbook. Nursing staff rely on the library to have current holdings of books in their particular specialization such as palliative care and medical-surgical nursing. These specialized books are only available in a hospital library. Public libraries do not buy them.

Currently, it is not popular to advocate for print resources. In this age of electronic access, it almost makes one look backward or regressive. I have even heard from librarians who say a patron will sometimes apologize for preferring a printed book, when they know the library has the electronic version. Nevertheless, ebook subscriptions are growing and more print books are becoming digitized and having both is good.

For 38 years, librarians relied on The Brandon-Hill list of books and journals to help them make purchasing decisions for libraries, large or small. The list was first published in 1965 and in 2003 ended with the retirement of Dorothy Hill. Some medical librarians now rely on Doody Enterprises for the Doody's Core Titles, which like the Brandon-Hill, contains essential purchase recommendations. Finally, other libraries will not lend their reference books to other libraries. This may also include other books that may be expensive or too valuable to lend. So, if a library does not have a set of core book titles, the staff will be forced to go to another library and this sometimes means they will go without because of time constraints.

Journal purchasing

Journal subscriptions can be a more daunting task. There was a time when there were only print journals. In the beginning, a print subscription entitled the library to the online access at no additional cost. Very soon, the electronic journal was separated from the subscription and the librarian had to decide whether to buy the print or the electronic journal or both. Today, the choice is even more challenging because many of the online journals may not contain exactly what comes in the print and the print may have information that is not published online.

Each year, the librarian creates a list of journal titles for the next year's subscription. The list basically stays the same except for any changes that would cause one to reconsider a subscription. For example, copyright allows you to borrow up to five articles from one journal title, dated within the current 5 years. Borrowing more than five requires that you purchase a subscription. Also, price could become an issue or changes in the number of years of access. Sometimes a journal is "embargoed," which means that you could get access to 5 years except for the current year, or some other restriction in years of access. These are things the librarian must watch for and negotiate when purchasing journals. Also, the journal could become available in a database you subscribe to, making it unnecessary to get a separate subscription. The librarian's job is to know where each title is available so as not to spend money unnecessarily.

Database purchasing

There are different types of databases and your decisions on which one to buy will depend on your particular hospital research programs and staff needs. This is one of the benefits of having a librarian. He or she keeps up with the ongoing stream of new and changing electronic resources. There are numerous databases that claim to be "point-of-care," meaning that they aim to provide easier access to answers to questions. Some databases focus on evidence-based content. You may purchase a database that is particular to the Radiology Service or the Pathology Department in the hospital.

Nursing databases are focused on the particular topics and questions nurses deal with on a daily basis. There are several nursing databases; some more evidence based than others. It is your job to investigate all of these and compare content and pricing and ease of use. Even better is to get the nurses to use the databases and decide which one they prefer. Attending yearly meetings at regional and national conferences is a good way to keep up with the changes. Your institution should help with the costs of going to these meetings, but if that is not possible, I think it is still worthwhile to at least go for a couple of days.

Market research

The solo healthcare librarian constantly looks into new resources. One of the best ways to conduct research on products is to go to conferences. It helps to have hundreds of vendors all in one place, where you can compare products and ask questions. Ever since I saw the film, "The Big Kahuna" with Kevin Spacey, I think of his words that went something like "we become the hands of the company, shaking all the other hands." When you talk to vendors and publishers, you are representing your hospital staff needs. Scheuing (1998) talks about value-added purchasing. He says "By far the most powerful evolutionary force in the changing role of purchasing, however, has been the shift in focus from price to cost and on to value" (p. 3). He asks what will the purchase contribute to the organization's performance? This is an important question to keep in mind when selecting any resource.

Part of market research is trying things out before you buy. You can agree to schedule a trial of a product, which means the publisher will allow usage for a period of time at no charge. Here is where networking with other librarians is important. If you are able to join a local consortium of libraries, many times vendors are invited to a meeting in order to present their product to the group. The consortium can negotiate cost saving subscription deals for the member libraries. For example, a subscription that would normally cost $120,000 can be purchased for $30,000 as a consortium member.

The library's ROI

> "ROI is broken. Phew, there, I've said it."
>
> *(Winston, 2014, p. 167)*

In the book, *The Big Pivot: Radically Practical Strategies for a Hotter, Scarcer, and More Open World,* Andrew Winston speaks of major issues for business today. One of the Big Pivot strategies is to redefine ROI (return on investment). Winston says "... most companies use ROI as a blunt tool without measuring the full spectrum of value.... ROI and its close cousin, internal rate of return (IRR), have migrated from being useful decision-making aids to being mental straitjackets" (p. 167).

When hospital administrators look at the library budget, it is understandable that the expensive online resources require a justification or proof of their value. Medical information resources constitute a complex array of databases, electronic journals, electronic books, CDs and DVDs, and other packages owned by healthcare publishers and vendors. Studies have been conducted to assess the value of library purchases and one in particular comes to mind.

The Children's Healthcare of Atlanta, Georgia librarians conducted a cost−benefit analysis using an online tool provided by the National Network of Libraries of Medicine (NNLM). Their online usage statistics for 2008 showed that 25,134 articles were read by employees (Daniels, 2010). They chose a modest price of $25.00 per article, which is what a person would pay without having a library. There are some journals that charge twice this amount for one article. Plugging this information into the NNLM tool brought up a price for the read articles at $628,350. The library had spent $227,377 for both the print and electronic journals, thus a savings of approximately $400,000. The librarians also calculated the savings provided by having a library and librarian to conduct interlibrary loans. Overall, it was clear that it would cost much more not to have a library and librarians (Daniels, 2010). Of course, this is just the monetary expenses and savings. There are substantial, difficult to measure valuables such as time saved by employees and increased knowledge and efficiency in work.

Maintaining electronic resources

4

Chapter Outline Head

E-resources life cycle

In the previous chapter, we discussed briefly the purchasing of books and journals and other electronic resources. Maintaining the electronic resources is a major job sitting in the wheelbarrow. To give you a better idea of what this entails, here is a diagram created by Ebsco Publishing.

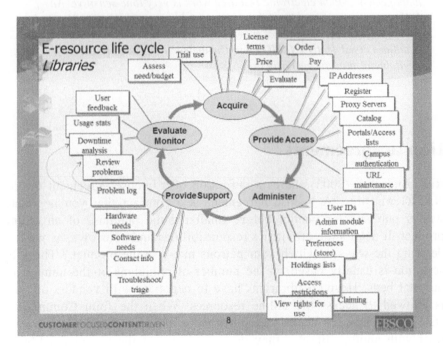

A solo healthcare librarian wears many hats. This one is titled the Electronic Resources Librarian or ERL. The North American Serials Interest Group, Inc. (NASIG, http://www.nasig.org) published the NASIG Core Competencies for ERLs in 2013. NASIG explains that the ERL is not an entry-level position. It is hard to imagine a librarian taking on a solo librarian position without knowledge of the E-resource life cycle. In a large library, there may be several librarians with each one assigned to a portion of the cycle.

The solo librarian ERL moves across the many sections involved in the cycle. It is interesting that NASIG also notes the need for flexibility in this crucial position. Here are some of the NASIG listed desired qualities for the ERL.

> *Flexibility, open-mindedness and the ability to function in a dynamic, rapidly changing environment. Flexibility is a crucial cognitive and affective attribute that operates on multiple levels. Within a single day an ERL may prioritize between various shifting tasks ... the ERL needs to be responsive to changing systems and user needs ... A high level of tolerance for complexity and ambiguity ... Unrelenting customer service focus and dogged persistence in the service of users ... Skillful time management. Much electronic resource work is very time-sensitive. An ERL must demonstrate the ability to plan and manage their own time and work assignments, and that of supervised staff, in order to make and meet deadlines consistently (NASIG Core Competencies Task Force, 2013), available at http://www.nasig.org.*

License agreements

Rick Anderson (2005) shares a definition of a license agreement on the NASIG website. "A license agreement is a contract that you negotiate with a publisher or vendor before finalizing the purchase of an online product. It details the provider's responsibilities and your own, as well as defining the ways in which your patrons may use the product." The subscription is usually based on the number of clinicians or the number of hospital beds. Hospital librarians have to negotiate with vendors on who is allowed to access the online resources. When the Joint Commission states that a hospital doesn't have to have a library, but only have a contract with another library, they don't realize that the contracted library does not purchase additional access in their license agreement for the affiliated hospital staff. It would be cost prohibitive. Therefore, many doctors and other clinical staff can be shut out of online access to needed information at affiliated hospital libraries. They may be able to use their library, but still have no online access to the medical literature. Depending on where you work and your institution's size and number of employees, negotiations will vary, so there is no point in going further in this area.

Jobbers

Jobbers is what librarians call the companies that provide the service of ordering your list of journals from the various publishers. Of course you pay the jobber to do this, but it is well worth the money because of the time saved for you. Jobbers also take care of any claims that come up. Let's say you have a list of 100 journals and each month as you are check-ing them in, as they arrive by mail, or even better, your volunteer notices as he or she is checking them in, that last month's issue is missing for a particular journal. This is when the jobber takes on the job of contacting the publisher for you. You submit a "claim" and they do the rest. They also contact publishers when online access is not working. Today, it is probably more the case that the library has very few print subscriptions and mostly online journals.

E-resources summary

Overall, the e-resources cycle begins with assessing the budget for the next year. Sometimes you decide to renew a contract, sometimes you go with another resource. You may do a trial period where patrons can use the prod-uct for a limited amount of time. Before deciding to purchase, careful scru-tiny is given to all license agreements. Next, the orders go in and you create careful documentation and records. The Information Technology department is notified and given the URL for them to post on the library website. Throughout the year, the URL must be checked to make sure you have online access. This is something your volunteer may be able to do, although patrons are very quick to let you know when they cannot access their favor-ite journal. There is also the job of maintaining a holdings list of all titles of journals. Knowing which titles are in what databases or available through a separate subscription, or knowing what years are covered in each subscrip-tion is essential to insuring no duplicate purchasing occurs. One other main-tenance job, not mentioned in the e-cycle graph, is updating the library's holdings in the Docline online interlibrary loan database. Entering new journal titles and removing titles or editing the years held of a particular title is important for interlibrary lending to run smoothly. When a hospital doesn't have books or journals to place on Docline, as a reciprocal borrower/lender, the hospital cannot participate in Docline. This entire cycle begins again the next year. For any questions about the e-resources life cycle, you can always contact another librarian. Again, networking with local library groups, regional, or national can put you in touch with knowledgeable librarians who are always willing to help.

All-around support

Chapter Outline Head

Support in the hospital

It appears that the support that librarians need most is from the hospital administrators. Today it is difficult for the administrators to see the value of the library and librarian. To be fair, they really can't be faulted because there are several ingrained mindsets operating here.

I used to think that the reason for the closing of libraries was due to a meme circulating among hospital administrators. The word "meme" was coined by Richard Dawkins in his book *The Selfish Gene*. Memes are like genes in the sense that they want to survive. They want to spread. Just as genes are instructions for making proteins, memes are instructions for carrying out behaviors. The idea that libraries and librarians are not needed because everything is free and on the Internet, is the worst kind of meme. Memes don't have to be true, they just have to be catchy. They spread because they appear to provide some kind of benefit or advantage even when they don't. Though this meme may contribute to the closing of libraries, I now have a broader perspective based on the earlier discussion in the "Evidence-Based Practice" section.

Part of this broader perspective includes thoughts from Shumaker (2012). I'm beginning to see that no matter how valuable something is, it is the perception in people's minds that makes it so. The words library and librarian carry a strong mindset and this causes me to consider adopting a title change to "Informationist." Administrators relate to the word library in the traditional manner based on the last 100 years. Shumaker (2012) points out that the common approach to communicating the value of the library has been based on quantitative data. How many books are checked out, how many reference interviews, how many interlibrary loans, and how many times are people accessing journals and databases. Though statistics are useful, there are more important elements that are usually overlooked. Shumaker says the passion for counting continues today when it comes to libraries. In addition, corporations are looking at measuring value and this means accountability and proof of value. It is no surprise that if the focus is on measuring usage of library materials and the numbers are down, the library appears expendable. Here is where value becomes critical and why I think a new informationist title, or embedded librarian may be in order.

Shumaker suggests that moving toward embedded librarianship has an important advantage. He gives a couple of examples and following his lead, I'd like to add a couple of my own. For example, if a patron gains critical knowledge by accessing a book in the library, or from an online database purchased by the librarian, will the librarian know about this? Shumaker says it is possible, but probably not because there is no system in place for this to happen. If a doctor or nurse gets help from the librarian with a search and decides to change their choice of therapy or treatment, again the librarian will know, but administrators will not. Shumaker says that when the embedded librarian works on a team, he or she gets immediate feedback and the managers of the team members also see the impact of the librarian's contribution. Overall, Shumaker makes the case that "the embedded librarian is in a much stronger position to demonstrate value than is the traditional practitioner of library services" (2012, p. 35).

This is another reason why networking is important. When you work with a committee, your service is witnessed by others. You may be aware and gratified by your contributions to your patrons' information needs, but if no one knows about it, you will personify the person who checks out books. If the reader is thinking about entering healthcare librarianship, be aware that this profession is in dynamic flux. Networking may be the operative word as we reimagine our profession. We have the technology which is already synonymous with networking. What is lagging behind is the perception of the librarian as limited and tied to the library. It is no surprise that the Johns Hopkins Welch librarians opted to disconnect from the library, but I will say more on this later.

Healthcare librarians have been networking with other librarians nationwide and have created amazing services. It is time for hospitals to tap this resource and put it to work to support evidence-based medicine, patient safety, prevention of diagnostic error, the creation of guidelines, research, and more. There are so many ways a librarian can contribute. If the reader is in need of ideas on how librarians can collaborate in the hospital setting, check out an excellent book by Dudden (2004) *Using Benchmarking, Needs*

Assessment, Quality Improvement, Outcome Measurement, and Library Standards. In addition to many practical tools for measuring the value of the library, Dudden provides a rich assortment of skills that are very helpful for the solo librarian.

Moreover, in this new age of electronic resources and evidence-based practice, it is the healthcare librarian's responsibility to offer service even when others may not think they need help. It is a moral and ethical responsibility to seek out ways to aid patrons who may not have the time or skills to find the information they need.

A supportive boss

Let it suffice to say that when you have a boss who "gets it," who knows the value of the library and librarian, it is wonderful! A supportive boss knows that a solo healthcare librarian is supporting the mission of the hospital by providing valuable information to various service lines in the hospital. He or she knows about the time-consuming jobs of purchasing and maintenance of the electronic resources. He or she also knows that where libraries that employ two or three librarians can have time to do many projects, a solo librarian's time is somewhat limited. For example, instead of a regular schedule of teaching classes, the solo librarian may opt to teach small groups when needed. Still, if your boss should decide that you should attend Morning Report, you will make the time, as that would be a priority.

Volunteers

The voices on the MedLib listserv strongly agreed they relied heavily on volunteers. Many of the jobs like shelving books, creating signage for the library, and checking the links to the online journals are best done by a volunteer. It takes time to train, but it is time well spent.

Support outside the hospital

Next to the ability to multitask and prioritize, networking was the most often given advice from the librarians who responded to my question on the MedLib Listserv. Words such as find a community for support, seek out others in person and online and build a strong network of librarians were offered.

There are local, regional, and national networks of medical librarians. If you do not have a local consortium, you can begin with the National

Network of Libraries of Medicine (NN/LM) with its eight regions in the United States. The NN/LM mission statement is available on their website at http://nnlm.gov/. Basically, NN/LM is dedicated to supporting librarians and making biomedical information available throughout the United States to enable people to make informed decisions about their health. Attending regional meetings will provide you with not only friendships and librarians you can contact for help but also education and opportunities to meet vendors and keep up with changes in the publishing world. Nationally, you can join the Medical Library Association (MLA) and again, have support from a larger group of librarians who come from around the world. As already mentioned, joining the MedLib Listserv will put you in touch with knowledgeable librarians within and outside the United States.

Self-support

When we think of self-support, we often think of self-help books. The best self-help books for the medical librarian, in my opinion, are books that will increase your knowledge in your work. This includes courses and any other educational opportunities. This is one profession where constant learning is the norm. When you join the MLA, you will be able to take online classes, when available, and likewise NN/LM offers classes.

There are also ongoing educational pursuits that don't end. For example, you can always look for ways to improve your searching skills. You may want to join the listserv for expert searchers. There may come a time when you have a very challenging search and these librarians are happy to assist with their tips. Educate yourself on how to read medical literature. There is a series of papers written by Trisha Greenhalgh that will help you decipher papers written about economic analysis, drug trials, diagnostic or screening tests, statistics for nonstatisticians and more. These are available in the *British Medical Journal*. Put aside the cataloging and take time to read the latest issue of the *Journal of the American Medical Association (JAMA)* or the *New England Journal of Medicine (NEJM)*.

It almost goes without saying that it is important to take breaks. Sitting in front of a computer for a long time can be a strain on the eyes and we all know that sitting too long is not so good for your health. Just remember to get up and walk. Get out of the library. This is a good way to encounter a patron and remind them of the library services.

Afterthoughts

6

Chapter Outline Head

Remodeling the wheelbarrow

As discussed earlier, the body of biomedical literature continues to grow and with it the gap between evidence and practice. We have looked at the mindsets and the pervading culture of hospitals and doctors. At the same time, there is the inexplicable closing of libraries with medical librarians disappearing from hospitals. In an editorial by Klein-Fedyshin, she warns that without a qualified librarian to support a collection of books and journals, and to conduct searches or deliver articles when needed, the quality of care will be diminished (2010). At a time when the Affordable Care Act, Medicare and the Institute of Medicine are looking at ways to improve healthcare delivery, it seems counteractive to not be utilizing healthcare librarians. The editorial makes the point that insurance providers count the number of tests, surgeries, and drugs administered, but no one measures the level of knowledge brought to the care. Klein-Fedyshin foresees a time in the future where healthcare institutions will score their "information readiness" in a similar way that we now score "most wired hospitals." When care of patients varies significantly from doctor to doctor and hospital to hospital, some patients may not be receiving the best care due to a lack of needed information.

Finally, I must say something more about any title changes for librarians. The Johns Hopkins movement to embedding informationists is commendable and also may result in the undervaluing of the many existing healthcare librarians. There, I 've said it. Understandably, some changes begin with small pioneering steps and perhaps this is intended as such. To return to Davidoff's argument for a better medical information delivery system, I have to agree that we are in desperate need of revision. However, wouldn't it make sense to utilize the existing medical librarians throughout the country and recruit more people to the profession, rather than creating informationists or embedded librarians as replacements? The contention may be that the healthcare librarian today does not have the proper background education for working on a team with clinical staff. I believe this argument is groundless.

The existing healthcare librarians are quite capable of locating the needed information without having as much knowledge as the doctor. They are capable of locating pertinent information no matter the subject. They are also capable of writing up a synthesis of the information, when needed. I don't think it is necessary for the librarian to analyze and interpret the medical statistics. Many of us have trouble deciphering the medical literature statistics. Greenhalgh (2010) in Chapter 5, *Statistics for the Nonstatistician*, explains "In this age where medicine leans increasingly on mathematics, no clinician can afford to leave the statistical aspects of a paper entirely to the 'expert'. If, like me, you believe yourself to be innumerate, remember that you do not need to be able to build a car in order to drive one" (p. 61). Librarians understand that when the doctor reads the literature, he/she can determine whether there should be further analysis of the content in order to decide whether the information justifies changing a diagnosis or moving toward the creation of a new guideline.

What we need to develop is a partnership with healthcare librarians as part of the team. A team should have diverse knowledge and abilities. The medical librarian brings to the team, skill in searching and an intelligence to continue learning whatever the subject. Teamwork is sharing knowledge in order to produce something greater than the parts. Relationships and teamwork are built on trust and working together over time. It is probable that the librarian's knowledge of a medical subject would increase over time. No system is in place to test this, and I agree with Davidoff (2011) that it is time to build one. However, let's be careful that we're not tipping the wheelbarrow in a way that will displace or obsolesce the current population of healthcare librarians. Now, I must confess that in 2005 I responded to a comment in *The Lancet* by William Summerskill who suggested more studies to be done to evaluate the effectiveness of using clinical librarians. My vision at the time was of a program where healthcare librarians could earn additional certification as in the way nurses do and other allied healthcare staff. What I had in mind was the credentialed healthcare librarian conducting a search to provide literature to support a treatment or test performed on a patient, thus enabling the creation of a current procedural terminology (CPT) code under Evaluation and Management (E/M) and thus generating revenue for the hospital (Burns, 2005). What I didn't envision is what is happening with the movement toward informationists today. To be clear,

I think the idea of going outside the library and becoming more readily available to hospital staff is a good idea. What doesn't feel right is the perception created that those medical librarians who remain in the library are obsolete. On the other hand, the future of healthcare librarians looks promising when I read what Scott Plutchak writes.

Plutchak (2012) speaks about the "dawning of the great age of librarians." He places our profession within a much larger framework where we are part of the generation that people will talk about in the future as the people who shaped the future of libraries and librarians. What I like most is when he says:

> "... we can experiment like crazy. We do not have to worry about getting
> it "right"—we will never know. That will be determined by how the
> culture shapes itself over the next couple of hundred years. Undoubtedly,
> many of our experiments will go nowhere, will be seen to be dead ends
> and wrong turns" (2012, p. 18)

It is time for hospital administrators to capitalize on the benefits of having a healthcare librarian on the team. Of course, having a medical librarian is not a panacea. We know the state of healthcare is complex, but clearly, eliminating medical librarians is not going in the right direction. Whether librarians become informationists or some other arrangement develops, we may have to pivot again and again. The future role of the healthcare librarian is still in the formative stage. We need leaders with the vision to take us to the next platform for action.

References

Asch, D. (2014). Innovation in medical education. *New England Journal of Medicine*, *371*(9), 794−795.

Bastian, H. (2010). Seventy-Five trials and eleven systematic reviews a day: How will we ever keep up? *PLOS Medicine*, *7*(9). Available from: http://dx.doi.org/10.1371%2Fjournal.pmed.1000326.

Bennett, N. (2005). Family Physicians' information seeking behaviors: A survey comparison with other specialties. *BMC Med Inform Decis Mak*, *5*(9). Available from: http://dx.doi.org/10.1186%2F1472-6947-5-9.

Burns, E. (2005). Evidence-based searching. *The Lancet*, *366*(9490), 979−980.

Chevalier, J., & Gheerbrant, A. (1996). *Dictionary of symbols*. New York, NY: Penguin Group.

Cimino, J.J. (2013). Practical choices for infobutton customization: Experience from four sites. *AMIA, Annual Symposium Proceedings*, 2013 (ecollection 2013), 236−245.

Connor, E. (2007). *Evidence-based librarianship: Case studies and active learning exercises*. Oxford, UK: Chandos Publishing.

Daniels, K. (2010). Got Value? Journal collection analysis is worth the effort. *Medical Reference Services Quarterly*, *29*(3), 275−285.

Davidoff, F. (2000). The informationist: A new health profession? *Annals of Internal Medicine*, *132*(12), 996−998.

Davidoff, F. (2011). Deliverying clinical evidence where it's needed: Building an information system worthy of the profession. *Journal of the American Medical Association*, *305*(18), 1906−1907.

Dhaliwal, G. (2013). Known unknowns and unknown unknowns at the point of care. JAMA. *Internal Medicine*, *173*(21), 1959−1961.

Dudden, R. (2004). *Using benchmarking, needs assessment, quality improvement, outcome measurement, and library standards*. New York, NY: Neal-Schuman Publishers, Inc.

Eden, J., Wheatley, B., McNeil, B., & Sox, H. (2008). *Knowing what works in health care: A roadmap for the nation*. Washington, DC: The National Academies Press.

Feldman, S. (2004). *KM world*. Retrieved from The high cost of not finding information, <http://www.kmworld.com/Articles/PrintArticle.aspx?ArticleID=9534>.

Graber, M. L. (2014). The next organizational challenge: Finding and addressing diagnostic error. *The Joint Commission Journal on Quality and Patient Safety*, *40*(3), 102−110.

Green, M. L. (2000). Residents' medical Information needs in clinic: Are they being met? *The American Journal of Medicine*, *109*(3), 218−223.

Greenhalgh, T. (2010). *How to read a paper: The basics of evidence-based medicine*. Hoboken, NJ: Wiley-Blackwell.

Kolowich, S., (2010). Embedded librarians: Johns Hopkins ahead of curve. USA Today online at <http://www.usatoday.com>.

Maatta, S., & Wallmyr, G. (2010). Clinical librarians as facilitators of nurses' evidence-based practice. *Journal of Clinical Nursing, 19*(23–24), 3427–3434.

McGowan, J. H. (2008). Just-in-time information improved decision-making in primary care: A randomized controlled trial. *PLoS ONE, 3*(11), e3785. Available from: http://dx.doi.org/10.1371/journal.pone.0003785.

Newman-Toker, D. E., & Pronovost, P. J. (2009). Diagnostic errors: The next frontier for patient safety. *Journal of the American Medical Association, 301*(10), 1060–1062.

Plutchak, T. S. (2012). Breaking the barriers of time and space: The dawning of the great age of librarians. *Journal of the Medical Library Association, 100*(1), 10–19.

Rovner, J. (2014). *IOM wants big change in doc training*. Retrieved from Kaiser Health News, <http://www.medpagetoday.com/PublicHealthPolicy/MedicalEducation/46986>.

Sackett, D. L. (2000). *Evidence-based medicine*. New York, NY: Churchill Livingstone.

Scheuing, E. E. (1998). *Value-added purchasing*. Menlo Park, CA: Crisp Publications, Inc.

Shumaker, D. (2012). *The embedded librarian: Innovative strategies for taking knowledge where it's needed*. Medford, MA: Information Today, Inc.

Singh, H., Meyer, A. N., & Thomas, E. J. (2014). The frequency of diagnostic errors in outpatient care: Estimations from three large observational studies involving US adult populations. *BMJ Quality and Safety, 23*(9), 727–731.

Swennen, M. (2013). Doctors' perceptions and use of evidence-based medicine: A systematic review and thematic synthesis of qualitative studies. *Academic Medicine, 88*(9), 1384–1396.

Tanenbaum, S. J. (2009). Comparative effectiveness research: evidence-based medicine meets health care reform in the USA. *Journal of Evaluation in Clinical Practice, 15*(6), 976–980.

van Dijk, N. (2010). What are the barriers to residents' practicing evidence-based medicine? A systematic review. *Academic Medicine, 85*(7), 1163–1170.

Weaver, D. (2011). Enhancing resident morning report with "daily learning packages". *Medical Reference Services Quarterly, 30*(4), 402–410.

Winston, A. S. (2014). *The big pivot: Radically practical strategies for a hotter, scarcer, and more open world*. Boston, MA: Harvard Business Review Press.

Zipperer, L. (2010). *Newsletter of the hospital libraries section of the medical library association*. Retrieved from Medical Library Association, <http://hls.mlanet.org/wordpress/wp-content/uploads/2011/03/V34N3.pdf>.

Index